SINUS INFECTIONS

PROFESSIONAL GUIDES TO TREATING

SINUS INFECTIONS

DR. J. WALLER

Contents

INTRODUCTION

Common respiratory disorders called sinus infections, sometimes called sinusitis, are brought on by inflammation and swelling of the tissues lining the sinuses. The air-filled cavities that surround the eyes and nose are called sinuses. A sinus infection may arise when the normal flow of mucus is obstructed, either by bacterial or viral infection, allergies, or other causes.

Acute sinus infections are those that go away quickly, whereas chronic sinus infections last for a long time. Numerous symptoms, such as headaches, facial pain or pressure, nasal congestion, and a fullness in the face, can be brought on by the illness.

Effective management and alleviation from sinus infections require knowledge of the conditions' causes, signs, and remedies. Sinus infections may affect daily functioning, regardless of the cause—a cold, allergies, or other factors and prompt medical attention is typically essential for an accurate diagnosis and effective treatment.

CHAPTER ONE

Identifying Sinus Ailments

The swelling and inflammation of the sinus cavities, which are the hollow spaces behind the nose and eyes, is referred to medically as sinus infection or sinusitis. The mucous membrane lining these canals secretes mucus, which aids in the collection of dust, germs, and other airborne particles.

A blockage in the mucus's regular drainage can result in an accumulation of mucus and an environment that is favorable to the growth of bacteria or viruses, which can cause sinus infections. There are several potential causes of the obstruction, such as:

Viral Infections: Inflammation brought on by common cold or flu viruses might result in sinusitis.

Bacterial Infections: Although less often than viral ones, bacterial sinus infections can arise as a follow-up infection after a cold.

Allergies: Inflammation of the sinuses can result from allergic reactions to environmental factors such as dust, pollen, or pet dander.

Growths in the nasal passages that obstruct sinus drainage are known as nasal polyps.

Deviated Septum: Sinusitis may be exacerbated by an anatomical problem in the nasal cavity.

Sinusitis primarily comes in two forms:

Acute Sinusitis: Usually lasting a few days to a few weeks, acute sinusitis is frequently linked to upper respiratory infections or colds.

Chronic Sinusitis: This type of sinusitis lasts longer than 12 weeks and can be brought on by a number of conditions, such as nasal polyps, deviated septum, or recurrent infections.

Typical sinus infection symptoms include:

- congestion in the nose
- facial pressure or pain
- Headache
- blotchy nasal discharge
- Cough
- Weary
- Absence of scent

- a sore throat

Evaluation of the patient's symptoms, medical history, and occasionally imaging tests are necessary for the diagnosis and treatment of sinus infections. Aside from supportive treatments like rest, fluids, and warm compresses, management may involve drugs such as nasal corticosteroids, decongestants, and antibiotics for bacterial infections.

If symptoms intensify, last longer, or show indications of a more serious infection, you must consult a doctor. Appropriate diagnosis and management can help reduce sinusitis symptoms and avoid complications.

Why People Get Sinus Infections:

Numerous conditions that promote inflammation and blockage of the sinus cavities can result in sinus infections, often known as sinusitis. The most typical reasons consist of:

Most sinus infections are caused by viruses, and they frequently develop as side effects of the common cold or the flu. Viruses irritate the sinuses and prevent them from draining normally.

Bacterial Infections: After a viral illness, bacterial sinus infections can arise as a secondary infection. In the clogged sinuses, bacteria may multiply and cause a more serious and protracted infection.

Allergies: Reactions to airborne allergens, such as dust mites, pollen, or pet dander, can inflame the sinuses and aggravate sinusitis.

Nasal polyps: These tiny, benign growths in the nasal passageways have the ability to clog sinuses and interfere with their regular outflow.

Deviated Septum: When the nasal septum, which separates the nostrils, is asymmetrical, it can cause problems with sinus outflow.

Infections of the Respiratory system: Conditions affecting the respiratory system, such bronchitis, have the potential to cause inflammation to move to the sinuses.

Environmental Irritants: Sinus inflammation may result from exposure to environmental irritants such air pollution or cigarette smoke.

Immune System Deficiencies: People who have compromised immune systems are at a higher risk of developing chronic sinus infections.

Different Sinus Infection Types:

Acute Sinusitis: This kind of sinus infection usually follows a viral upper respiratory infection and lasts for a brief period of time. Facial pain, nasal congestion, and discolored nasal discharge are possible symptoms.

Chronic Sinusitis: Unlike acute episodes, symptoms of chronic sinusitis may be more subdued and last longer than 12 weeks. It may be brought on by things like nasal polyps, recurrent infections, or structural problems with the nasal cavity.

Subacute Sinusitis: Similar to acute and chronic sinusitis, subacute sinusitis lasts four to twelve weeks.

Multiple occurrences of acute sinusitis within a year are indicative of recurrent sinusitis.

Fungal Sinusitis: Although rarer, fungal infections can result in sinusitis, especially in those with weakened immune systems or underlying medical disorders.

Allergic Fungal Sinusitis (AFS): This kind of sinusitis is frequently accompanied by nasal polyps and is linked to allergic reactions to airborne fungi.

Appropriate treatment and management of a sinus infection depend on knowing the kind of infection and its underlying cause. The optimal course of action for treating symptoms and avoiding recurrence is determined by a medical evaluation that includes a detailed assessment of symptoms and occasionally imaging testing.

Signs and symptoms

The symptoms of sinus infections, often known as sinusitis, can vary widely in terms of intensity and length. There is considerable overlap between the symptoms and those of other respiratory illnesses or common colds. Typical sinus infection symptoms include:

Nasal Congestion: One of the main signs of sinusitis is a sense of stuffiness or obstruction in the nasal passages. Inflammation and mucus buildup could be the cause.

Face Pain or Pressure: The forehead, cheeks, or area surrounding the eyes are common places to experience pain or pressure. When bending over or making abrupt movements, the discomfort could get greater.

Headache: Sinus infections are frequently linked to headaches caused by sinus infections. Frequently, the forehead, temples, or the region surrounding the eyes are the sites of localized pain.

Discolored Nasal Discharge: The mucus that comes out of the nose can have a yellow or green hue and be thicker. An infection is present as shown by this color shift.

Coughing: If the sinus drainage is creating irritation in the throat, a chronic cough may arise.

Loss of Smell: Nose congestion and inflammation are major causes of anosmia, which is a diminished or total loss of smell.

Sore Throat: Postnasal drip can irritate and cause discomfort in the throat.

Fatigue: Having a sinus infection can be physically taxing, which contributes to an overall sense of exhaustion.

foul Breath: Halitosis, or foul breath, may be caused by a buildup of germs and mucus in the sinuses.

Fever: A low-grade fever is sometimes associated with sinus infections, especially when the infection is bacterial.

It's crucial to remember that each person's symptoms may differ, and not everyone who has a sinus infection will have them all. Furthermore, depending on whether the sinusitis is acute or chronic, other symptoms may occur.

It's critical to get medical help right away if symptoms increase, last longer, or are accompanied by a strong headache, a high fever, or changes in vision. Appropriate diagnosis and treatment can reduce sinus infection symptoms and avoid consequences.

Identification and Medical Assessment

Examining the patient's medical history, symptoms, and, in certain situations, further diagnostic testing are used in the diagnosis and medical evaluation of sinus infections. This is a summary of the procedure:

Clinical Assessment:

A medical professional will start by performing a comprehensive clinical assessment and inquiring about symptoms including headaches, facial pain or pressure, nasal congestion, and any changes in nasal discharge. They will also ask how long the symptoms have lasted and whether they have returned.

Health Background:

Giving a thorough medical history is crucial. The diagnostic approach benefits greatly from knowledge of prior sinusitis episodes, allergies, respiratory infections, and any pertinent occupational or environmental exposures.

Physical Assessment:

Inspection of the neck, face, and nasal passages may be part of a physical examination. The medical professional may check the interior of the nose with a nasal speculum to look for indications of inflammation, nasal polyps, or other anomalies.

Diagnostic Standards:

If the symptoms fit the recognized diagnostic criteria for sinusitis, the healthcare provider may utilize them to make the diagnosis. These requirements frequently include the type and duration of symptoms.

Imaging Research:

Imaging tests could be suggested in specific situations in order to see the sinuses and make sure the diagnosis is correct. Typical imaging techniques consist of:

CHAPTER TWO

X-rays: A basic sinus X-ray can give a general idea of the architecture of the sinuses.

Computed Tomography (CT) Scan: CT scans provide more precise images of the sinuses and are useful in determining whether structural defects, obstructions, or other variables are causing sinusitis.

Endoscopy of the nose:

A thin, flexible tube equipped with a light and camera is used during nasal endoscopy to view the sinuses and nasal passages. This can assist in locating nasal polyps and other problems.

Swab or Culture

A nasal discharge swab or culture may be performed if a bacterial infection is suspected in order to pinpoint the exact bacteria causing the ailment. This aids in figuring out the best course of antibiotic therapy.

Testing for Allergies:

Allergy testing may be advised to identify particular allergens if allergies are thought to be a contributing factor.

It's crucial to remember that clinical examination is the main method used to diagnose sinus infections; imaging tests are not always required. Additionally, depending on the type and length of symptoms, medical professionals may distinguish between bacterial and viral sinusitis.

Those with sinus infection symptoms are advised to seek a medical professional's advice for a thorough assessment. Appropriate therapy and early diagnosis can help reduce sinusitis symptoms and avoid complications.

Methods of Therapy

Treatment for sinus infections, often known as sinusitis, is contingent upon the underlying cause, which may be bacterial, viral, or associated with other variables. The following are typical methods of treating sinus infections:

Symptomatic Reduction:

Medications available without a prescription, like decongestants and analgesics (like ibuprofen, acetaminophen, or pseudoephedrine), help alleviate symptoms. Nasal sprays with decongestants can be used for momentary relief, but prolonged use can cause rebound congestion.

Saline Nasal Irrigation:

Using a saline spray or solution, nasal saline irrigation helps clear the nasal passages of mucus and allergens. It may be a useful method for clearing nasal congestion and facilitating better breathing.

Drinking plenty of water

Maintaining adequate hydration facilitates improved sinus outflow and thins mucus. It can help to consume a lot of water and other liquids.

Warm Compresses:

Warm compresses applied to the face may help relieve sinusitis-related facial pain or pressure. Warmth can ease discomfort and increase blood flow.

Relax:

Sufficient sleep enables the body to concentrate on healing. Leaning back and obtaining adequate rest can aid the immune system in combating the virus.

Corticosteroids Intranasal:

It may be necessary to give intranasal corticosteroid sprays, such as mometasone or fluticasone, to lessen nasal channel irritation. Both allergic and non-allergic types of sinusitis can benefit from these drugs.

Antibiotics:

A medical professional may recommend antibiotics to treat the particular germs causing the sinus infection if it is bacterial in nature. Even if symptoms subside before the antibiotic course is out, it's imperative to continue the entire term of treatment.

Anti-histamines:

It could be advised to use antihistamines to treat allergy symptoms and lessen inflammation if allergies are a factor in sinusitis.

Breathing in corticosteroids:

Sometimes doctors will prescribe inhaled corticosteroids, which are usually used for allergies or asthma, to treat airway inflammation.

Immunotherapy:

Immunotherapy, or allergy shots, may be used to desensitize the immune system to particular allergens in cases of chronic sinusitis caused by allergies.

Surgery:

Surgery could be suggested in cases of structural problems, nasal polyps, or other difficulties associated with recurrent or chronic sinusitis. Enhancing sinus outflow and addressing underlying issues can be achieved with endoscopic sinus surgery.

For a precise diagnosis and a suitable treatment plan, speaking with a healthcare provider is essential. Antibiotic resistance may result from self-diagnosis, overuse, and ineffectiveness of antibiotics in cases where the infection is viral. Severe or persistent symptoms should be the reason to see a doctor for additional assessment and advice on the best course of action.

DIY Solutions & Self-Treatment

While sinus infections frequently require medical attention, there are certain self-care and home treatments that can reduce symptoms and aid in the healing process. Here are a few efficient natural treatments for sinus infections at home:

Saline Nasal Irrigation:

To irrigate the nasal passages, use a saline solution or saline nasal spray. This facilitates drainage, lessens inflammation, and thins mucus.

Warm Compresses:

To relieve pressure and pain in the face, apply warm compresses. For approximately fifteen minutes, cover the afflicted areas with a warm, damp cloth.

Drinking plenty of water

Make sure you stay hydrated by consuming lots of water, herbal teas, and clear broths. Drinking enough water keeps mucus thin and promotes improved drainage.

Inhaling steam:

Breathe in steam to help clear your nasal passages. You can take a hot shower, use a humidifier, or use a basin of hot water. Steaming with a few drops of eucalyptus oil added can increase its efficacy.

Relax:

Get enough sleep so that your body can recuperate. The immune system fights the virus more successfully when you sleep.

Raise Your Head:

To keep your head raised as you sleep, raise the head of your bed or use additional pillows. This may lessen congestion in the sinuses.

Hot Foods:

Include items high in heat, such horseradish, hot peppers, and spicy soups, in your diet. These meals can encourage drainage and help unclog nasal passages.

Avoid Being Around Irritants:

Steer clear of environmental irritants that can exacerbate sinus issues, such as strong scents or cigarette smoke.

Neti Pot:

To clean out your nasal passages, use a neti pot filled with saline solution. To prevent issues, use distilled or sterile water and practice good hygiene.

Warm Seawater Rinse:

Warm saltwater gargling might help ease sore throats and lessen postnasal drip irritation.

Remain Warm and Wet:

Keep the areas where you live warm and damp. Add moisture to the air by using a humidifier, especially in chilly indoor spaces.

Counterfeit Medicines:

Painkillers and decongestants are examples of over-the-counter medications that may offer momentary comfort. Nonetheless, take these drugs as directed by the manufacturer, and if you have any questions, speak with a doctor.

It's crucial to remember that these natural therapies are only adjuncts to medical therapy; they should not be used in place of it. Seek medical attention from a professional for an accurate diagnosis and course of treatment if symptoms intensify, last longer, or indicate a more serious infection.

Complications and Knowing When to Get Help

Even though sinus infections are usually common and usually go away with the right care, problems can occasionally occur. It's critical to be aware of potential side effects and to get medical help if your illness doesn't get better or if you have severe symptoms. The following issues and indicators call for medical intervention:

Prolonged Sinusitis:

Chronic sinusitis may be diagnosed if the sinusitis does not improve after 12 weeks of treatment. More thorough diagnosis and treatment may be necessary for this type of sinusitis.

Periodic Sinusitis:

Even though sinusitis can be treated, recurrent bouts may point to an underlying problem that requires more research and care.

Prolonged or Severe Symptoms:

It's critical to get medical help if your symptoms such as a persistently high fever, a severe headache, or increased facial pain—are severe or linger longer than you anticipated.

CHAPTER THREE

Transmission of Infection:

It is possible for sinus infections to spread to neighboring structures, which might result in consequences like:

An infection that spreads to the eye socket and results in redness, swelling, and poor eye movement is known as orbital cellulitis.

Pupil buildup in the tissues surrounding the eye is known as a periorbital abscess.

Intracranial Complications: If the infection progresses to the brain, rare but dangerous side effects like meningitis or a brain abscess may appear.

Vision Shifts:

Any changes in vision, such blurry or double vision, should be assessed right away by a medical expert.

Excruciating Headache:

A medical assessment is necessary if an over-the-counter pain reliever does not treat a severe or persistent headache.

Stiffness in the neck:

A fever and stiffness in the neck may indicate meningitis, in which case immediate medical intervention is necessary.

Exacerbation of Respiratory Symptoms:

A more serious respiratory infection or complication may be indicated if you notice an aggravation in your respiratory symptoms, such as shortness of breath or chest pain.

Those with impaired immune systems:

People who have compromised immune systems as a result of HIV/AIDS, cancer, or immunosuppressive drugs are more vulnerable to problems and should get help as soon as possible.

Constantly Green or Bloody Emission:

A more serious infection or other underlying problems may be indicated by a consistently green or bloody nasal discharge, even though discolored discharge is typical with sinus infections.

It is best to speak with a healthcare provider if you have concerns or are unclear about the severity of your symptoms. Seeking medical attention as soon as possible will help avoid complications and guarantee that sinus infections are treated appropriately. Do not wait to seek emergency care if symptoms increase quickly or if there are indications of a serious infection.

Preventive Actions

By taking preventative steps, one can lessen the likelihood of getting a sinus infection and the frequency of repeated bouts. The following are some methods to avoid sinus infections:

Continue to Practice Good Hygiene:

To stop the spread of germs and viruses, wash your hands frequently with soap and water. Refrain from using unwashed hands to contact your face, particularly your lips, nose, or eyes.

Maintain Proper Hydration:

Sufficient hydration facilitates healthy nasal outflow and keeps mucus thin. Water is your best beverage throughout the day.

Employ humidifiers:

Install a humidifier in your home, particularly in the winter or during dry spells. Drying out of the nasal passages can be avoided by adding moisture to the air.

Steer clear of irritants:

Avoid environmental irritants that might aggravate the nasal passages and raise the risk of sinus infections, such as strong scents and cigarette smoke.

Handle Allergies:

If you have allergies, seek medical advice to determine and control allergens that could cause sinusitis. Allergen avoidance and allergy testing may be necessary for this.

Nasal Mist:

To maintain the nasal passages free and to flush out irritants, employ nasal saline irrigation on a regular basis. This may be especially helpful for people who frequently get sinus infections.

A well-rounded diet

Keep a diet full of nutritious grains, fruits, and vegetables that is well-balanced. Overall immune function is supported by a nutritious diet.

Control GERD:

In order to treat your gastroesophageal reflux disease (GERD), collaborate with your doctor. Stomach acid reflux disease (GERD) can aggravate sinusitis by rerouting stomach acid into the throat and nasal passages.

Prevent Using Decongestant Nasal Sprays Excessively:

Rebound congestion can result from using over-the-counter decongestant nasal sprays for extended periods of time.

Deal with structural problems:

To learn about possible procedures for structural abnormalities in the nasal passageways, such as a deviated septum, see an ear, nose, and throat (ENT) expert.

Control Your Stress:

Utilize stress-reduction strategies, such as yoga, meditation, or relaxation exercises, as stress can impair immunity and exacerbate disease.

Immunizations:

Maintain current immunizations, such as the yearly flu shot. The chance of developing subsequent bacterial sinusitis can be decreased by avoiding viral infections.

Frequent Workout:

Regular physical activity will help to maintain immune system and general health.

Refraining from Ill People:

Avoid close contact with sick people if at all possible to lower the chance of virus transmission.

Personalized preventative methods created in cooperation with a healthcare practitioner may be beneficial for those who have a history of recurrent sinus infections or who have underlying medical issues. Preventive measures can also include timely treatment of respiratory infections and routine medical examinations.

CONCLUSION

In summary, sinus infections, often known as sinusitis, are prevalent respiratory ailments that can be uncomfortable and interfere with day-to-day activities. Recurrent or chronic sinusitis may require more extensive therapy, even though the majority of cases are acute and remit with reasonable treatment.

For those seeking healing and trying to reduce the danger of further infections, it is essential to comprehend the causes, symptoms, and preventive actions. Key elements of preventative care include maintaining proper hygiene, drinking plenty of water, controlling allergies, and avoiding irritants in the surroundings.

It's critical that anyone suffering symptoms get medical help as soon as possible. A medical expert is able to accurately diagnose conditions, identify underlying causes, and suggest the best course of action, which may involve medication, nasal irrigation, or, in certain situations, surgery.

People can minimize the negative effects of sinus infections on their general health and preserve healthy sinus function by adopting preventive measures into their daily lives and promptly resolving symptoms. Proactive sinus health care involves regular communication with healthcare experts and knowledge of personal risk factors.

THE END